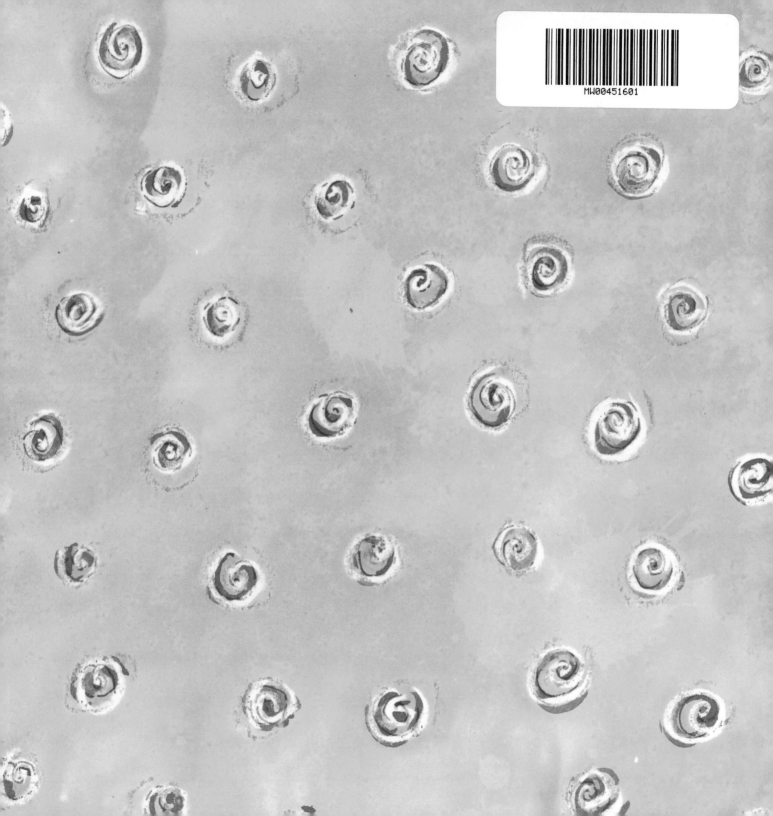

Text copyright © 2009 Carmen Martinez Jover
www.carmenmartinezjover.com
illustrations copyright © 2009 Rosemary Martinez
www.rmartdesign.com

ISBN 978-970-94103-2-7

A tiny itsy bitsy Gift of Life
1st edition, November 2005
2nd edition, March 2006
3rd edition, June 2009
4th edition, June 2011

Story: Carmen Martinez Jover
Design & illustrations: Rosemary Martinez
Layout: Victor Alfonso Nieto

Special thanks to Lone Hummelshoj, www.endometriosis.org
and Sandra de la Garza, www.ami-ac.com

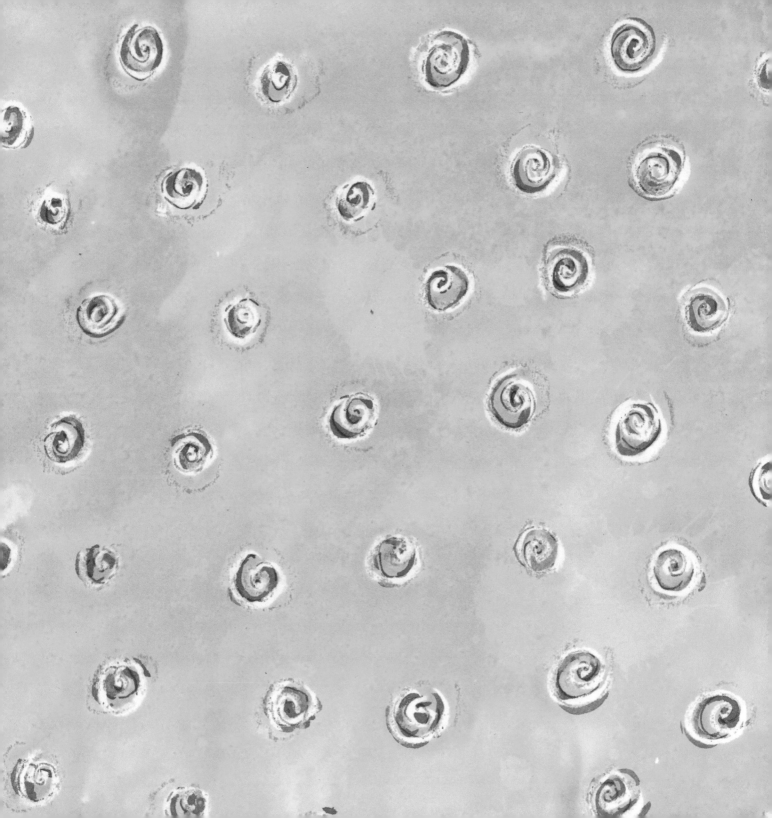

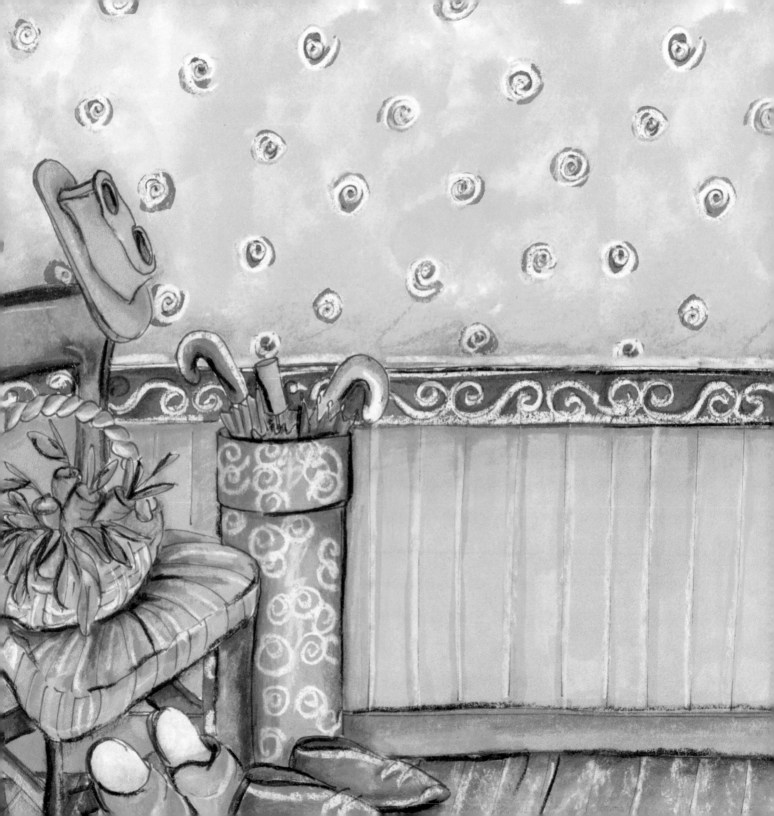

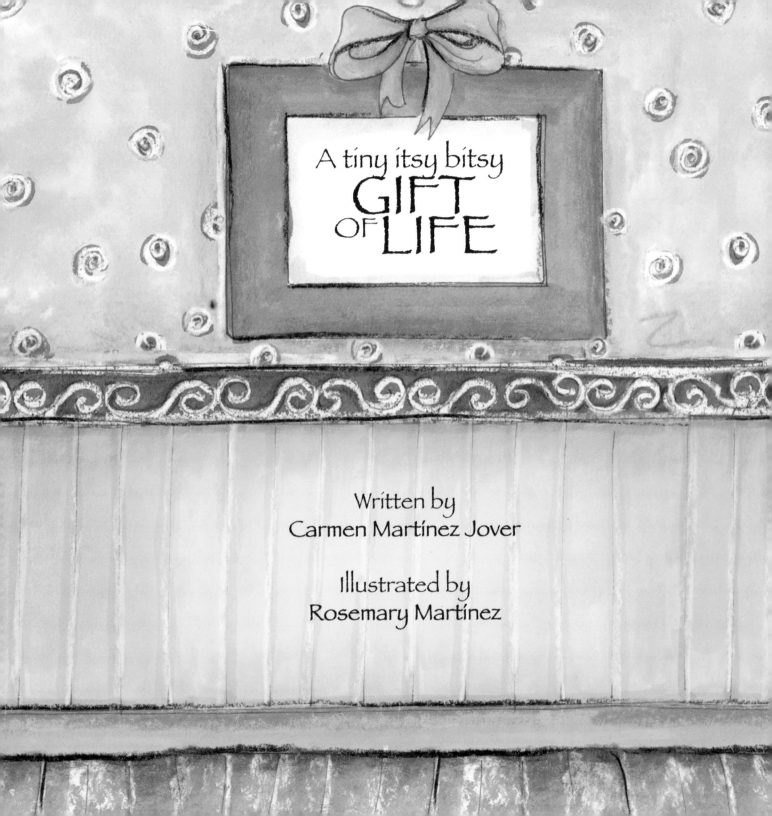

A tiny itsy bitsy
GIFT OF LIFE

Written by
Carmen Martínez Jover

Illustrated by
Rosemary Martínez

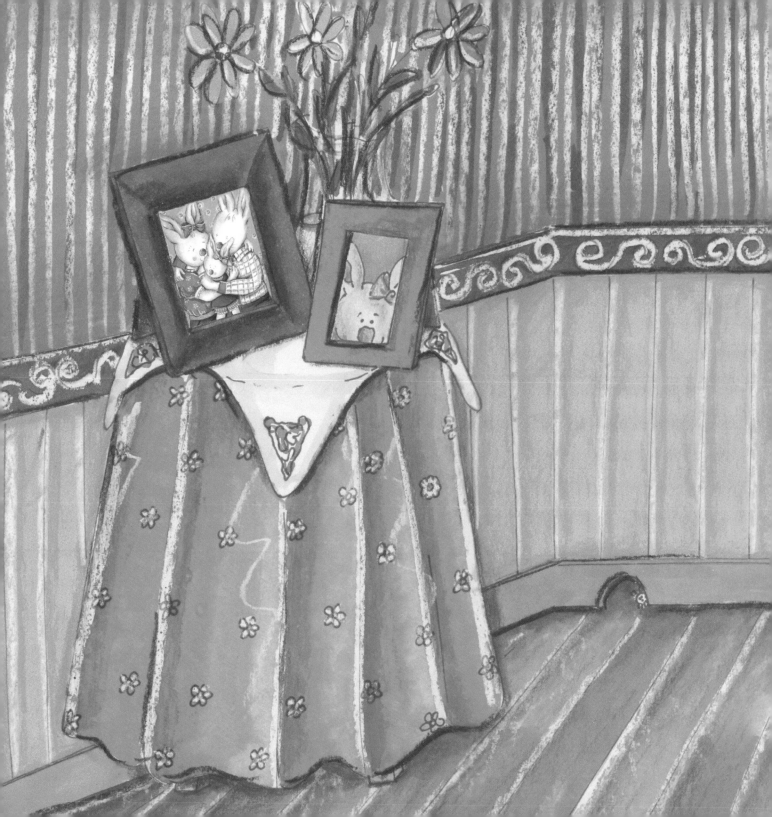

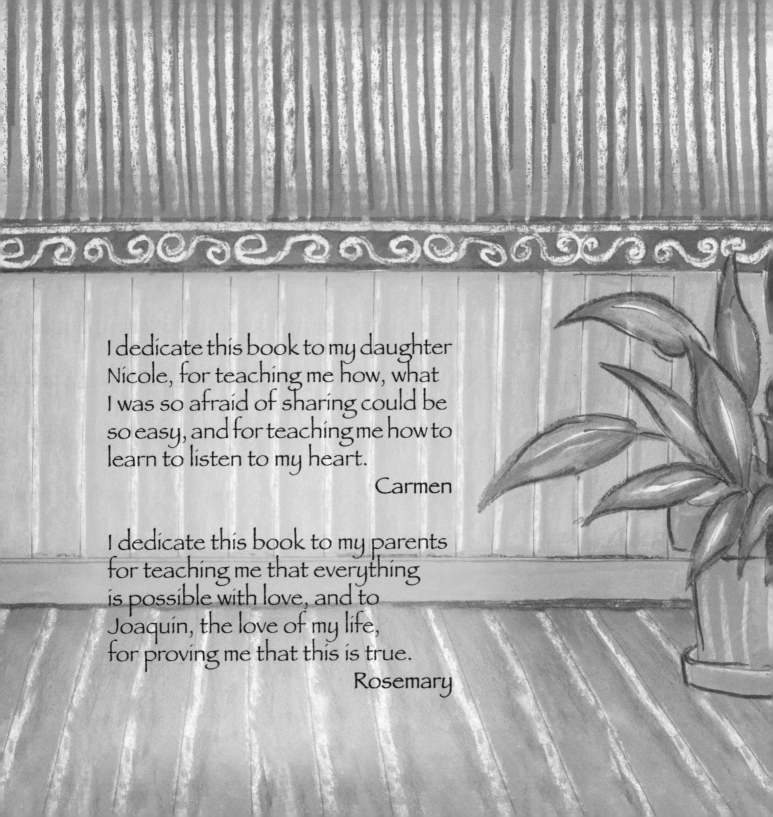

I dedicate this book to my daughter
Nicole, for teaching me how, what
I was so afraid of sharing could be
so easy, and for teaching me how to
learn to listen to my heart.

Carmen

I dedicate this book to my parents
for teaching me that everything
is possible with love, and to
Joaquin, the love of my life,
for proving me that this is true.

Rosemary

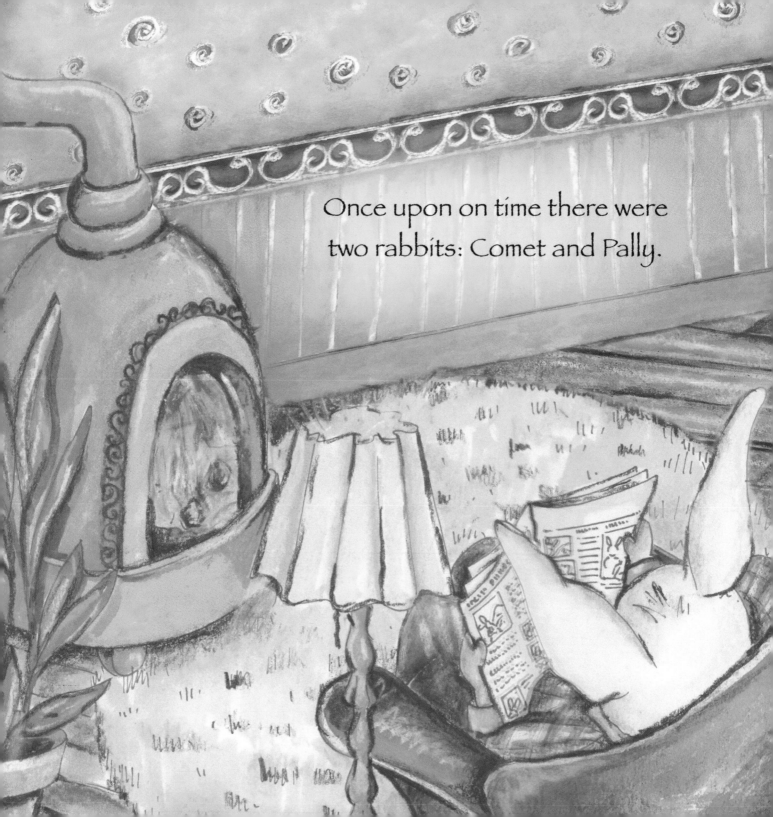

Once upon on time there were two rabbits: Comet and Pally.

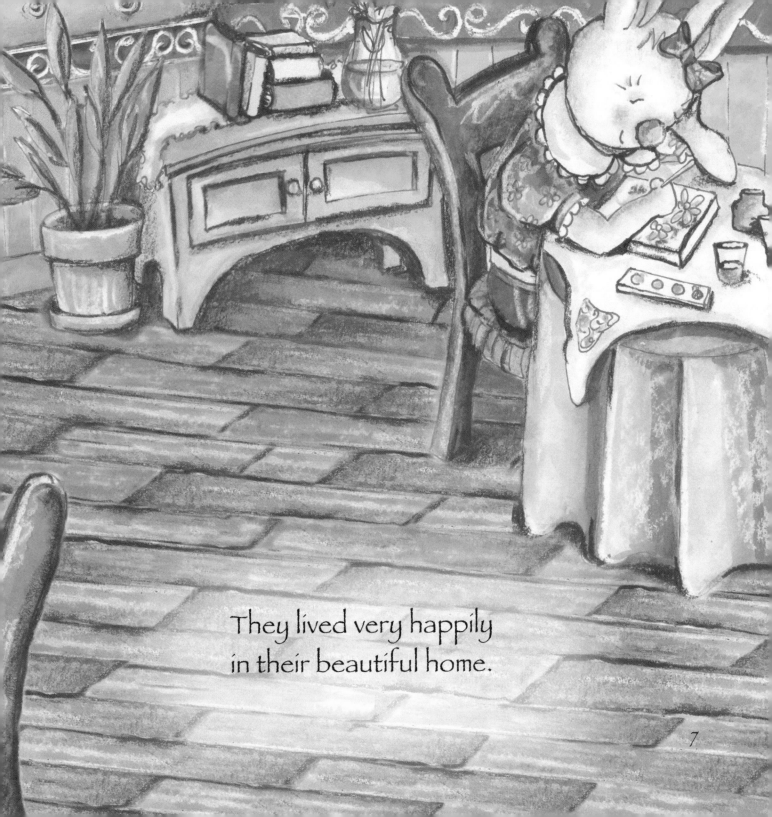

They lived very happily
in their beautiful home.

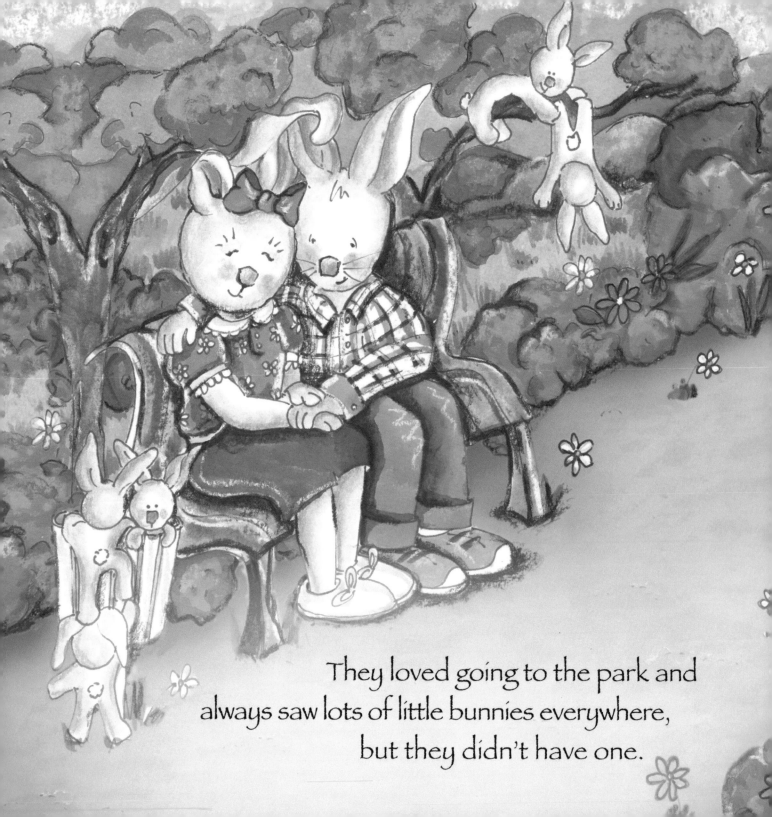

They loved going to the park and
always saw lots of little bunnies everywhere,
but they didn't have one.

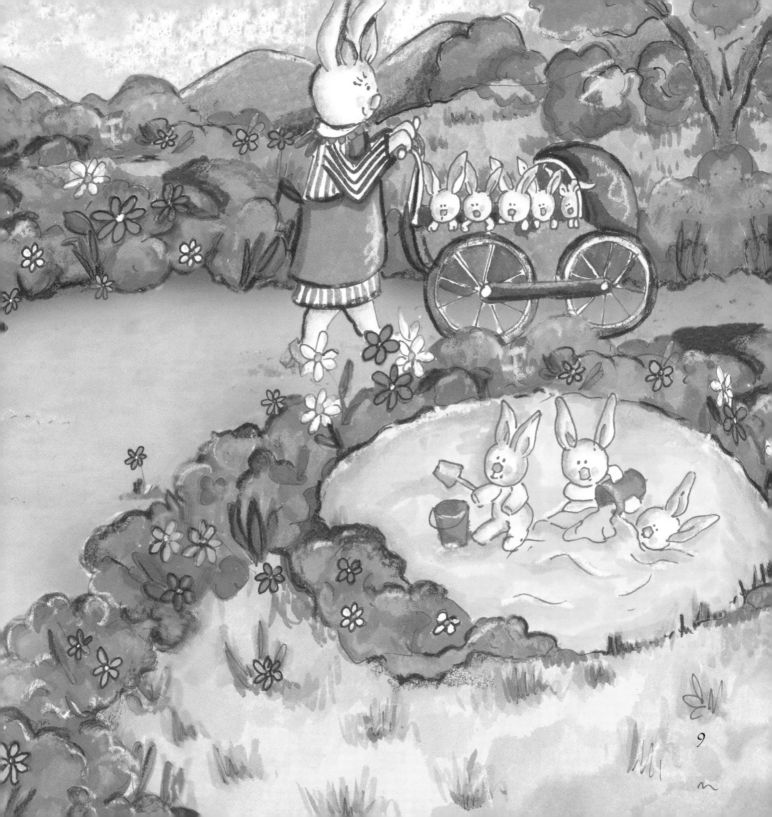

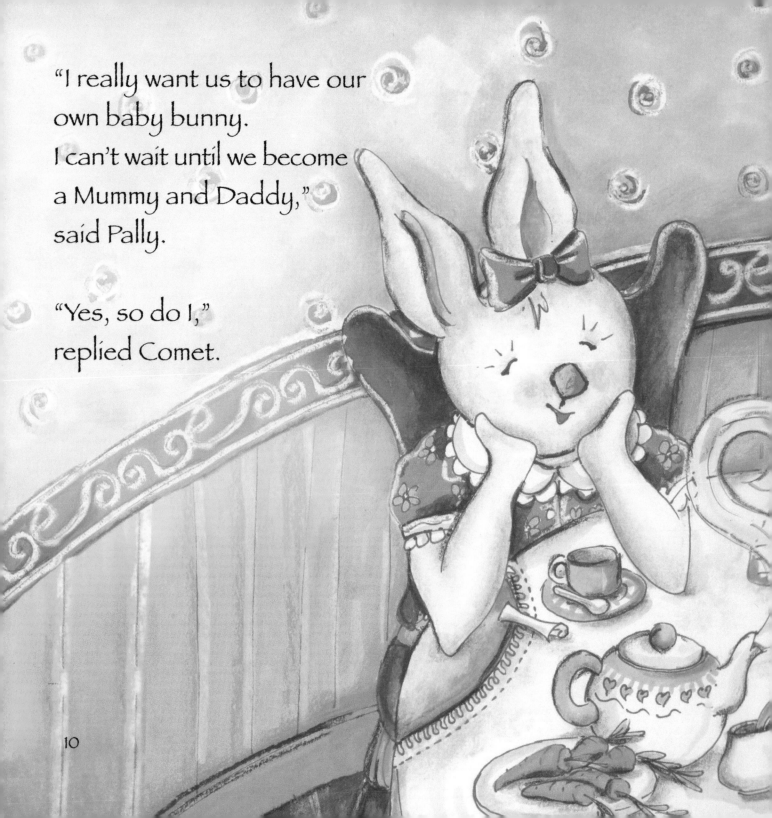

"I really want us to have our own baby bunny.
I can't wait until we become a Mummy and Daddy,"
said Pally.

"Yes, so do I,"
replied Comet.

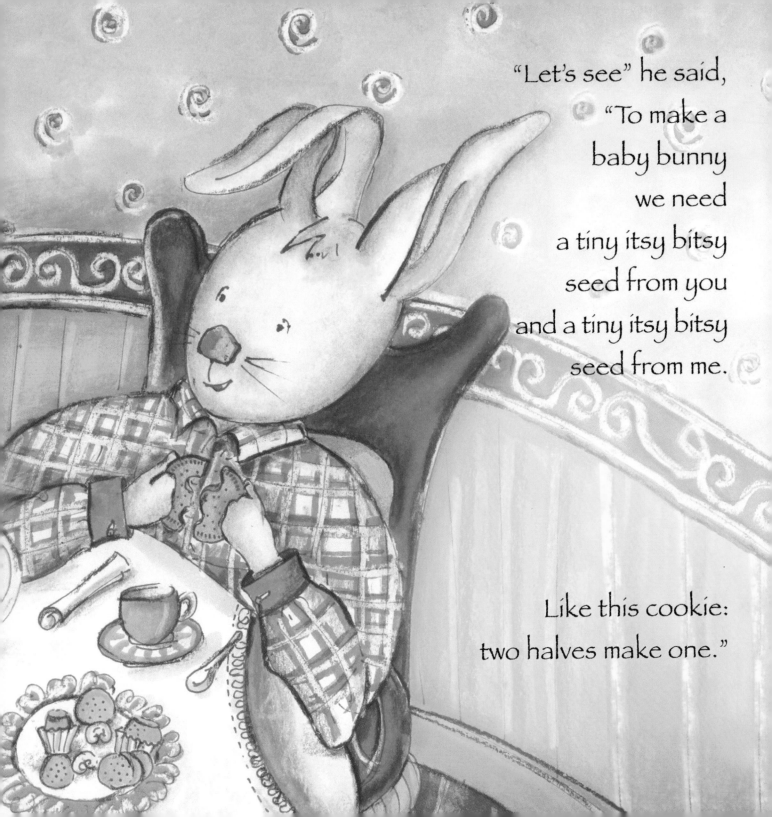

"Let's see" he said,
"To make a
baby bunny
we need
a tiny itsy bitsy
seed from you
and a tiny itsy bitsy
seed from me.

Like this cookie:
two halves make one."

But, Spring went by...

And Summer went by...

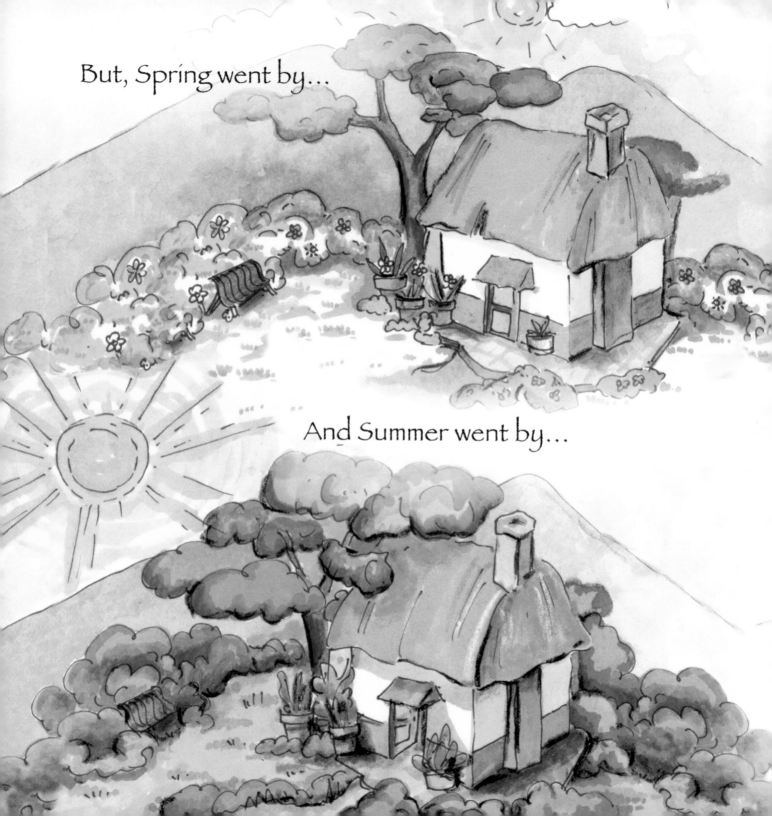

And Autumn went by...

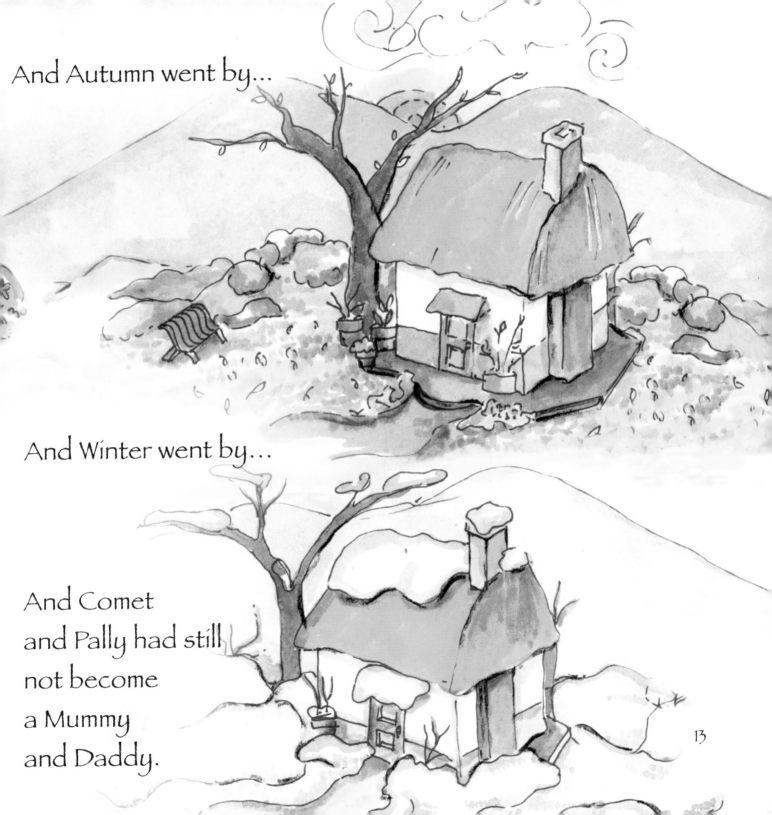

And Winter went by...

And Comet
and Pally had still
not become
a Mummy
and Daddy.

13

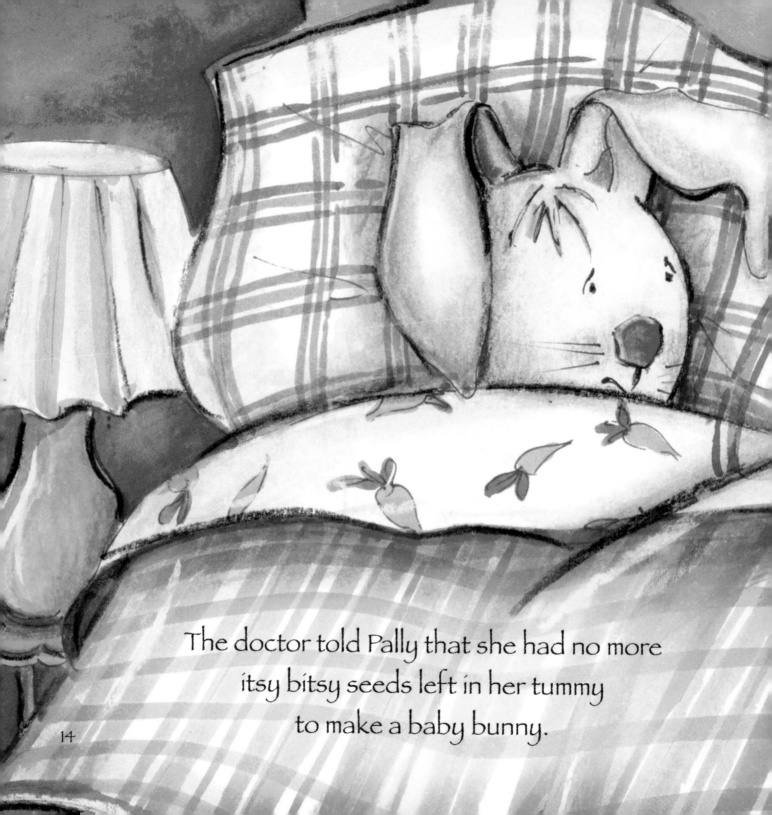

The doctor told Pally that she had no more
itsy bitsy seeds left in her tummy
to make a baby bunny.

14

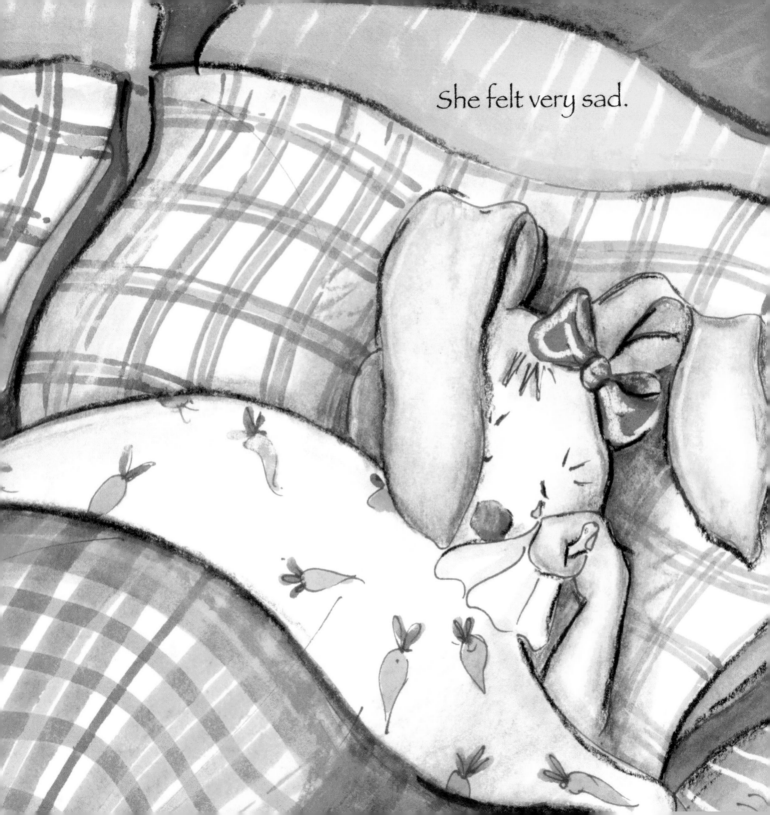

She felt very sad.

One special sunny day, a lady rabbit knocked on the door.

They had never seen her before.

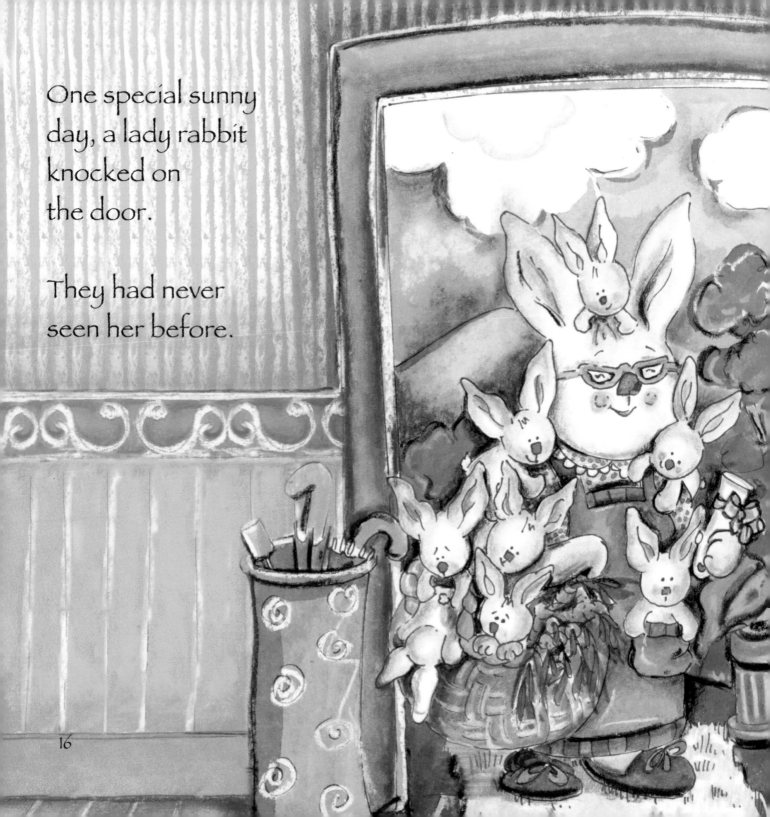

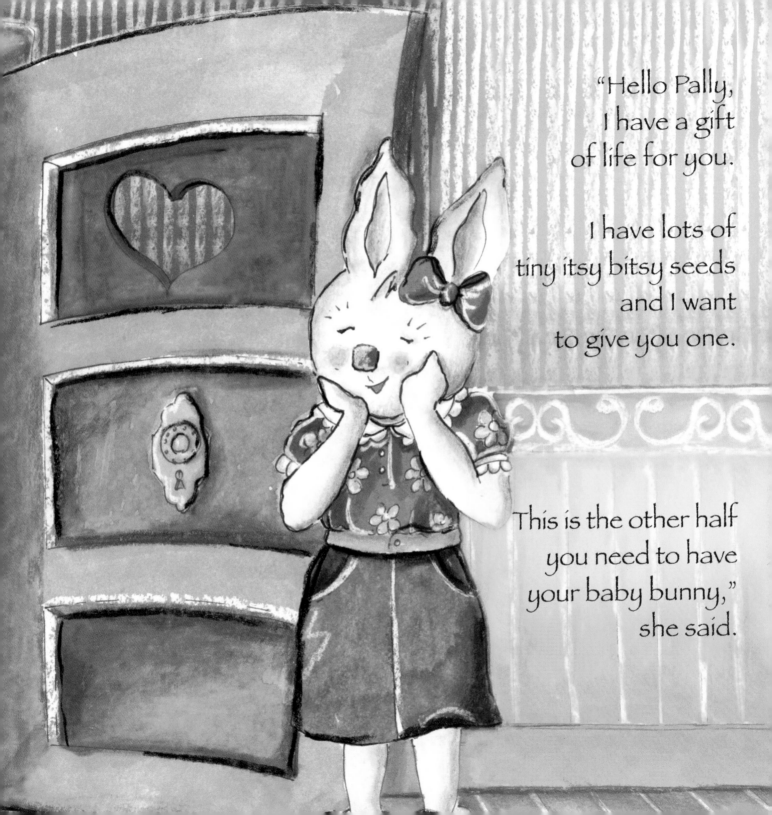

"Hello Pally,
I have a gift
of life for you.

I have lots of
tiny itsy bitsy seeds
and I want
to give you one.

This is the other half
you need to have
your baby bunny,"
she said.

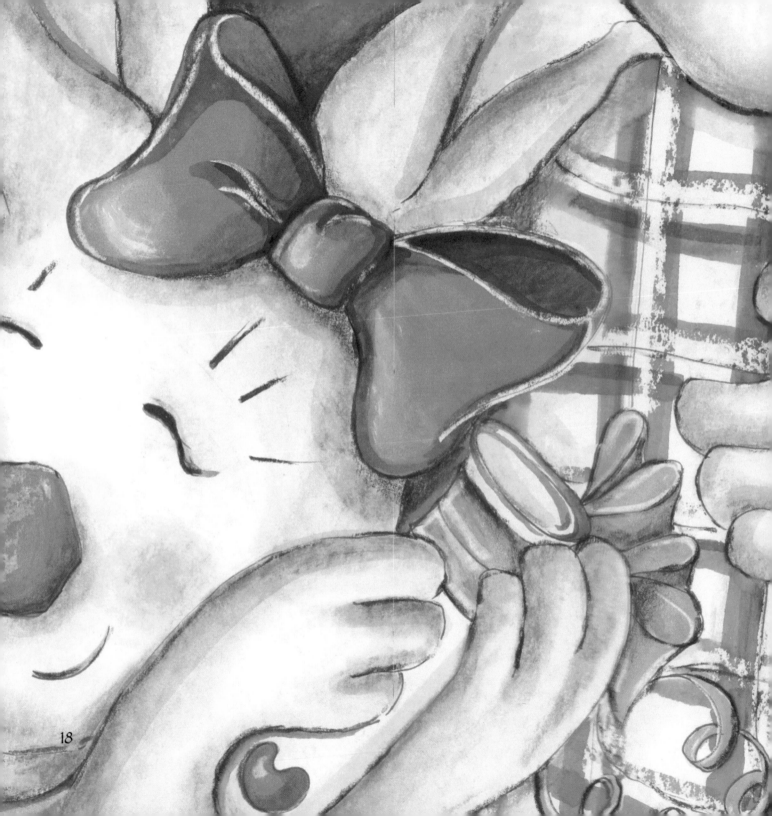

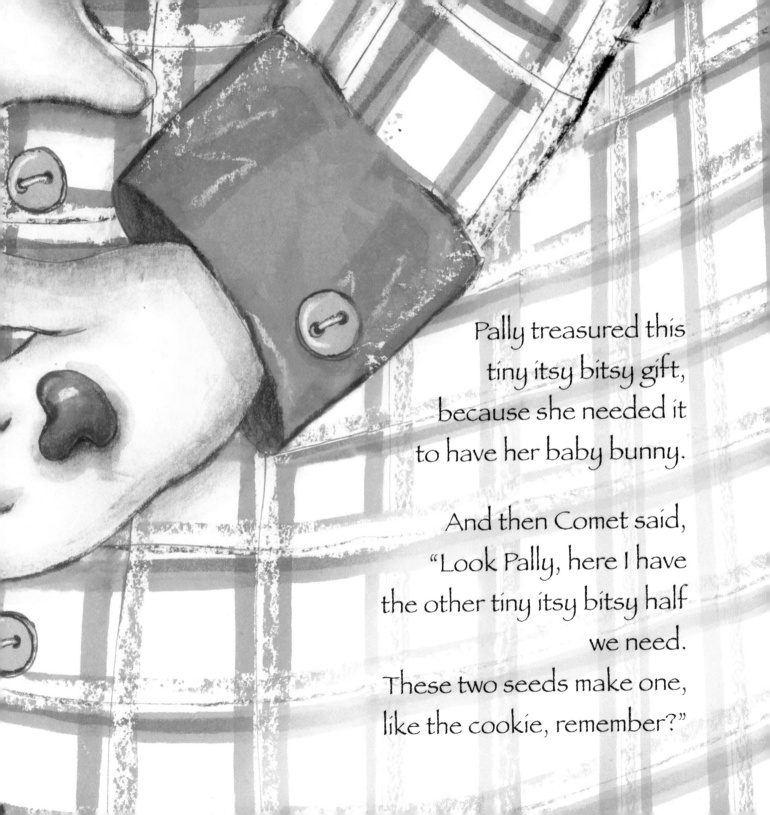

Pally treasured this
tiny itsy bitsy gift,
because she needed it
to have her baby bunny.

And then Comet said,
"Look Pally, here I have
the other tiny itsy bitsy half
we need.
These two seeds make one,
like the cookie, remember?"

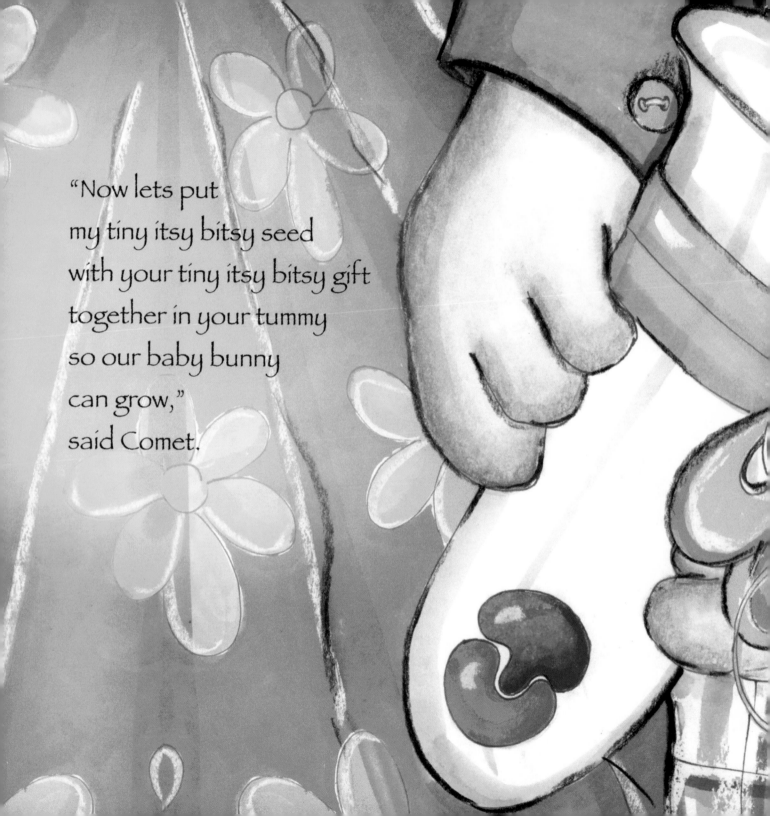

"Now lets put
my tiny itsy bitsy seed
with your tiny itsy bitsy gift
together in your tummy
so our baby bunny
can grow,"
said Comet.

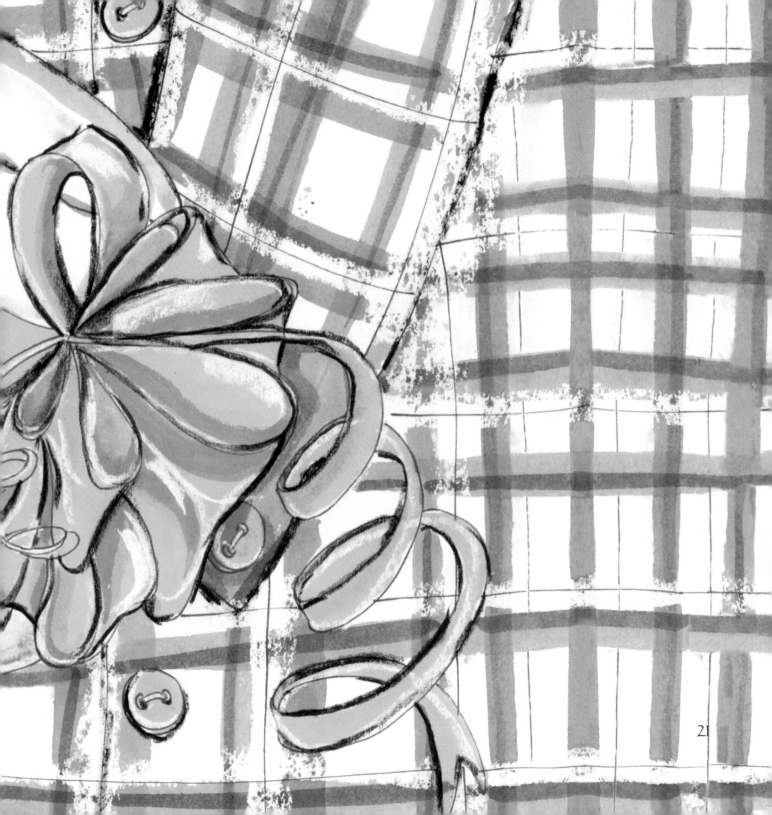

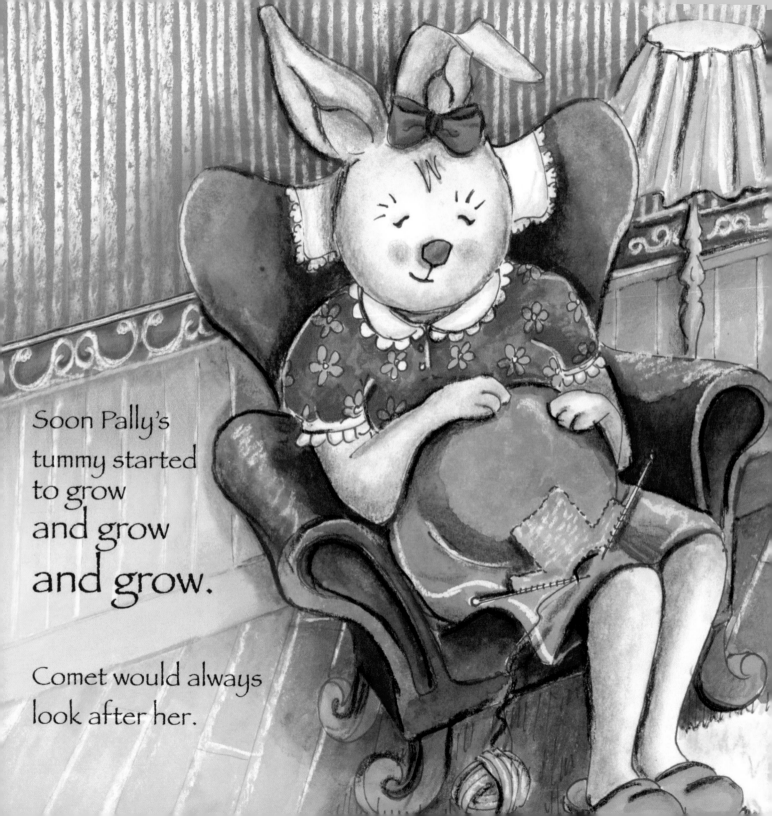

Soon Pally's
tummy started
to grow
and grow
and grow.

Comet would always
look after her.

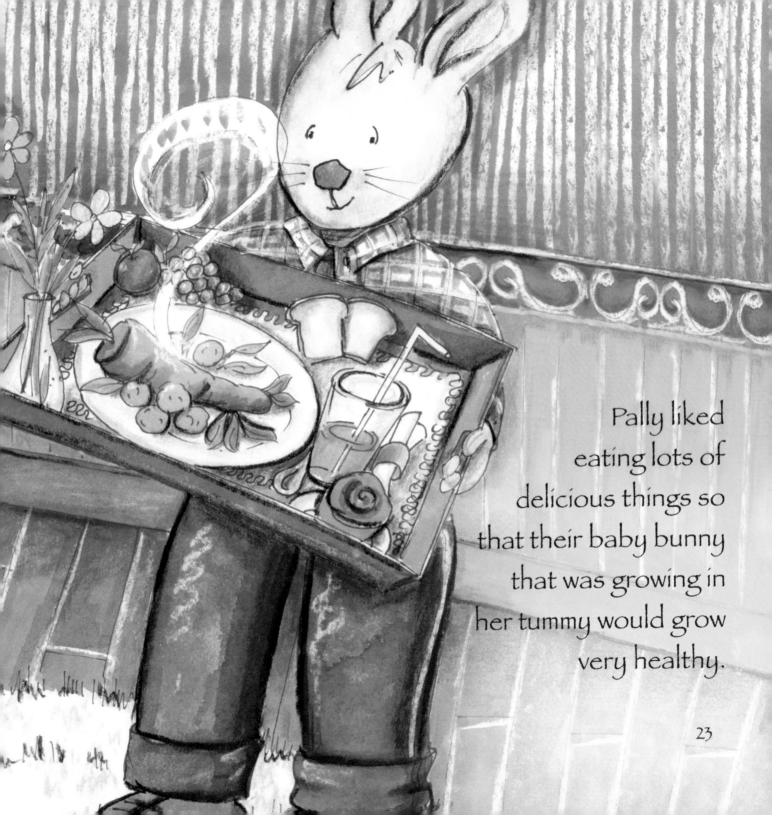

Pally liked eating lots of delicious things so that their baby bunny that was growing in her tummy would grow very healthy.

23

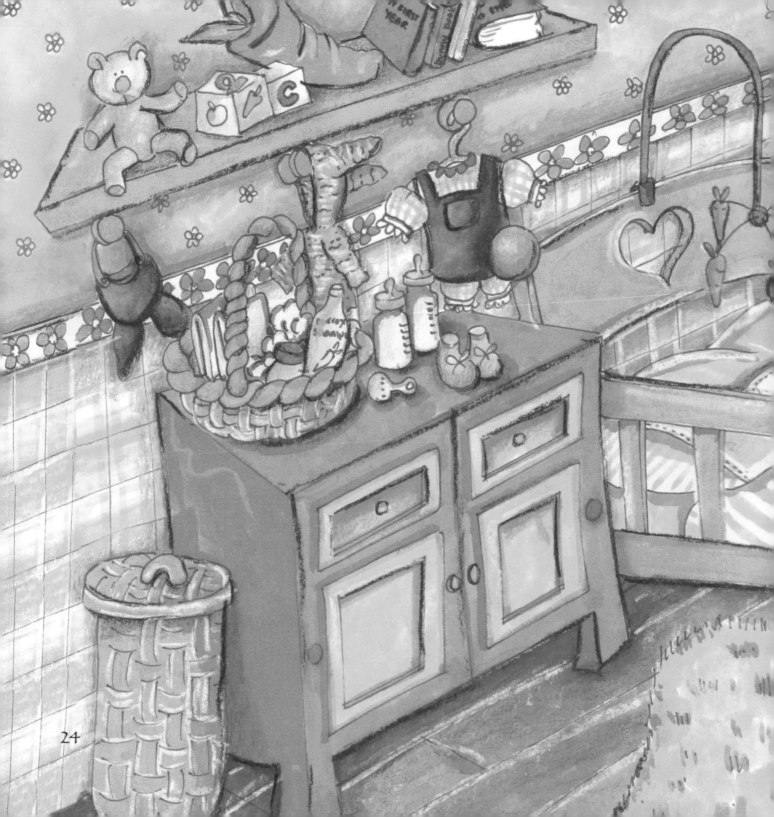

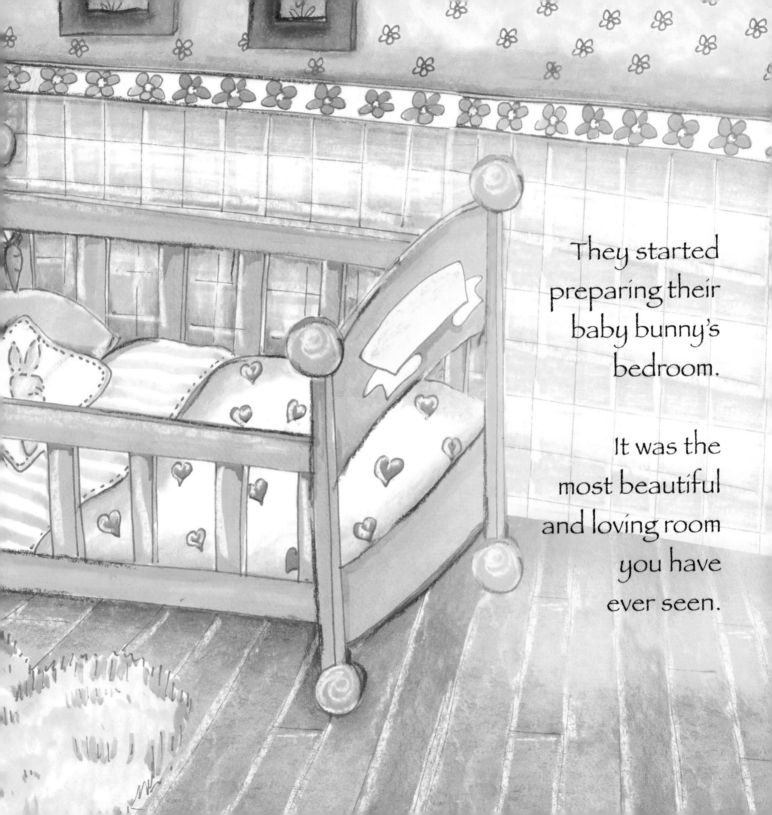

They started
preparing their
baby bunny's
bedroom.

It was the
most beautiful
and loving room
you have
ever seen.

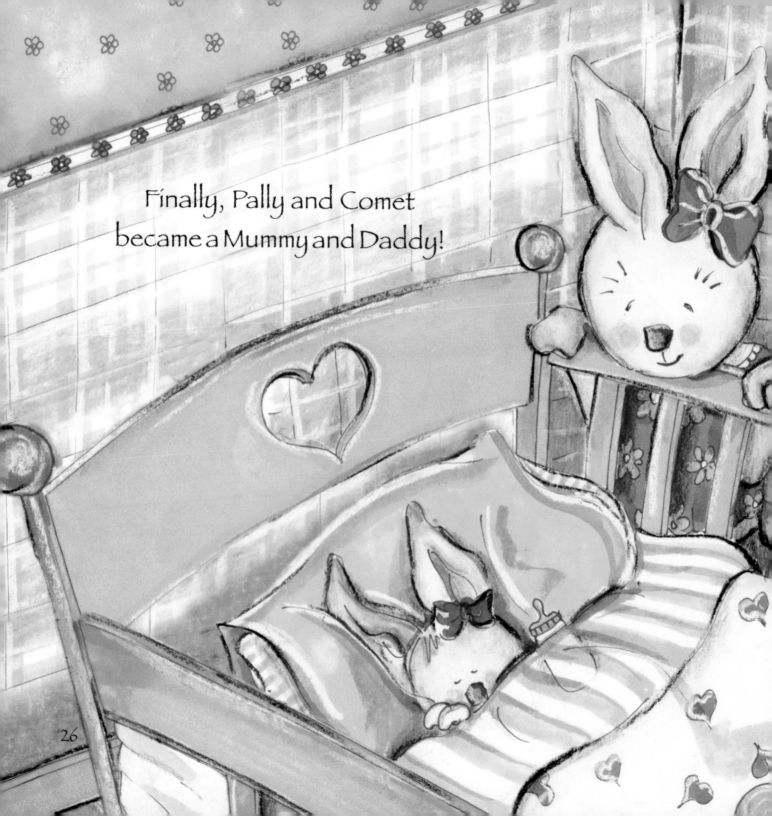

Finally, Pally and Comet
became a Mummy and Daddy!

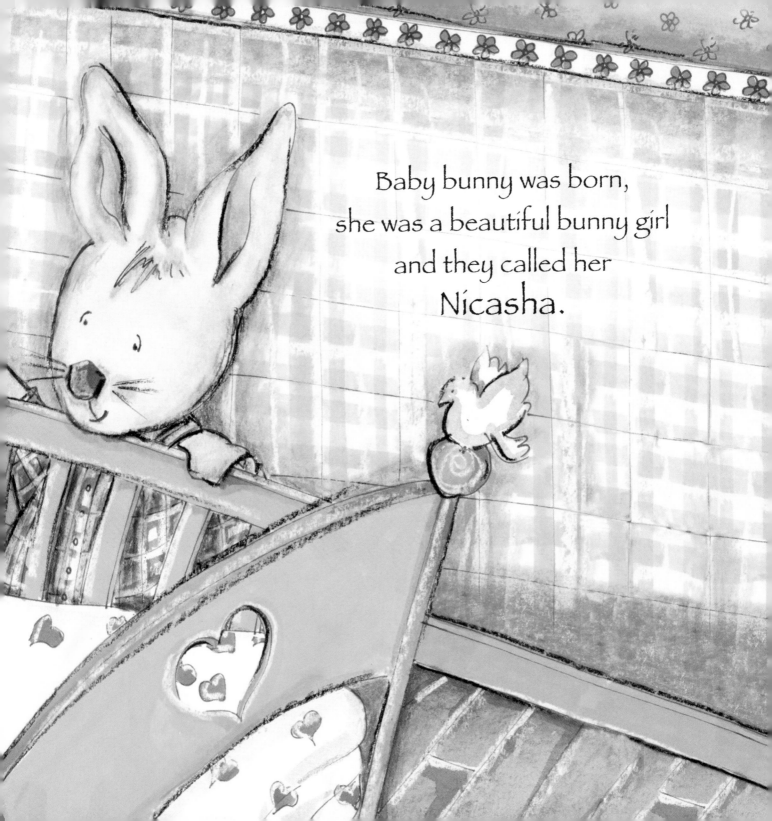

Baby bunny was born,
she was a beautiful bunny girl
and they called her
Nicasha.

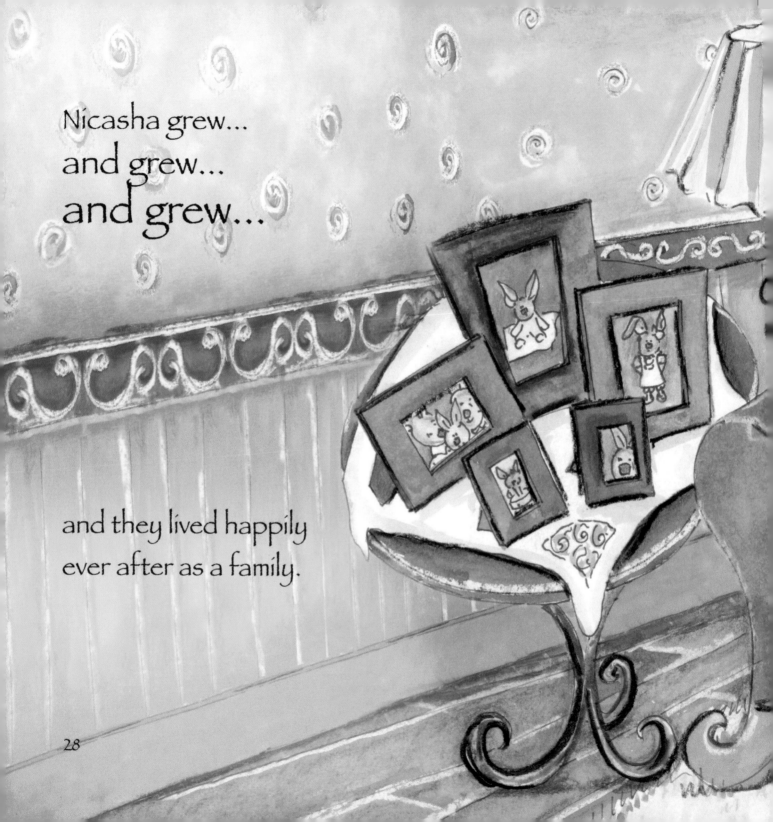

Nicasha grew...
and grew...
and grew...

and they lived happily
ever after as a family.

28

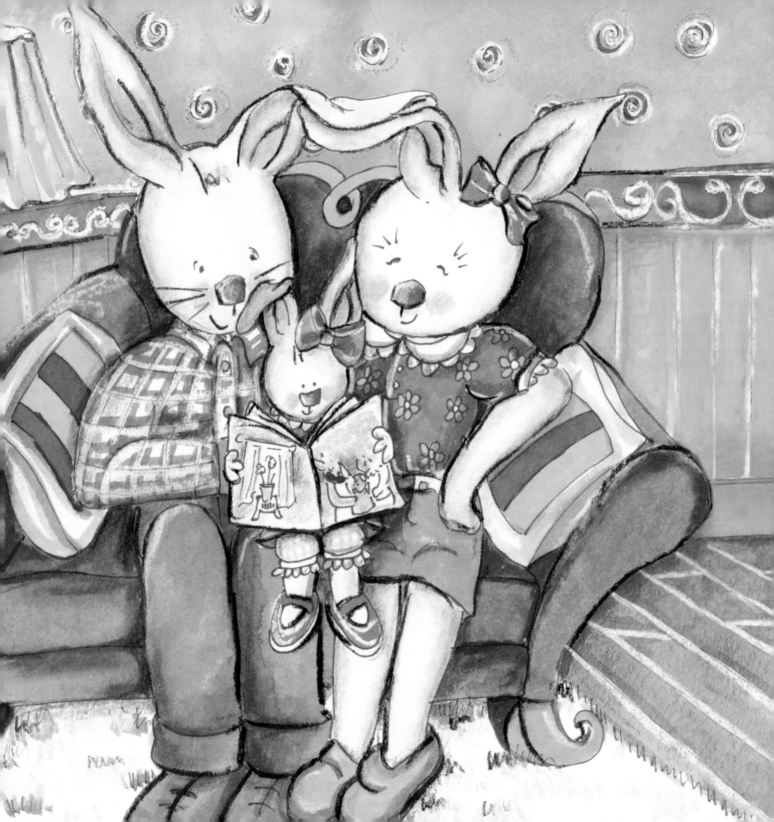

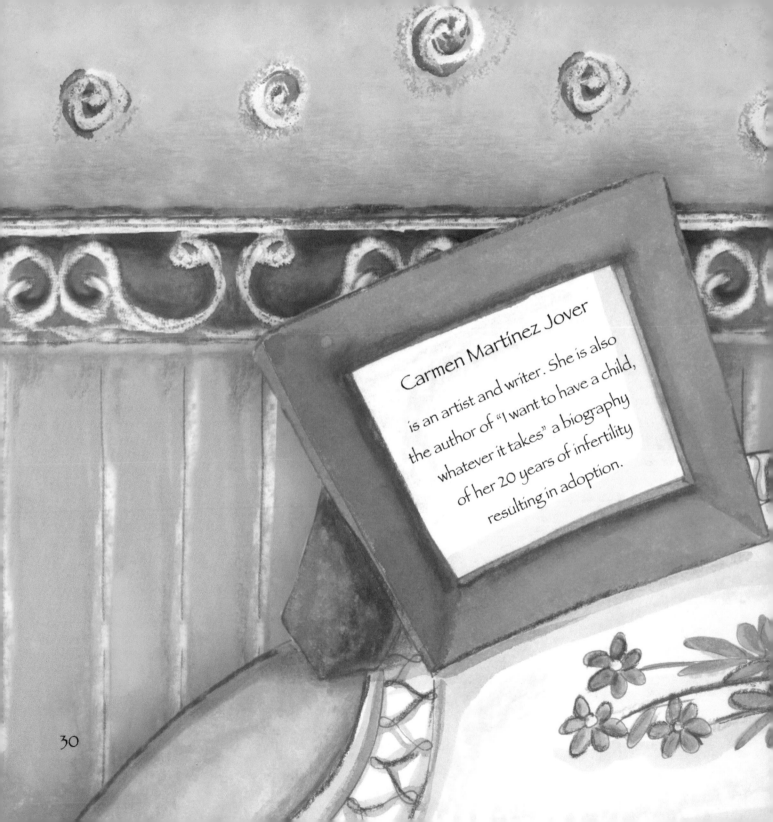

Carmen Martínez Jover

is an artist and writer. She is also the author of "I want to have a child, whatever it takes" a biography of her 20 years of infertility resulting in adoption.

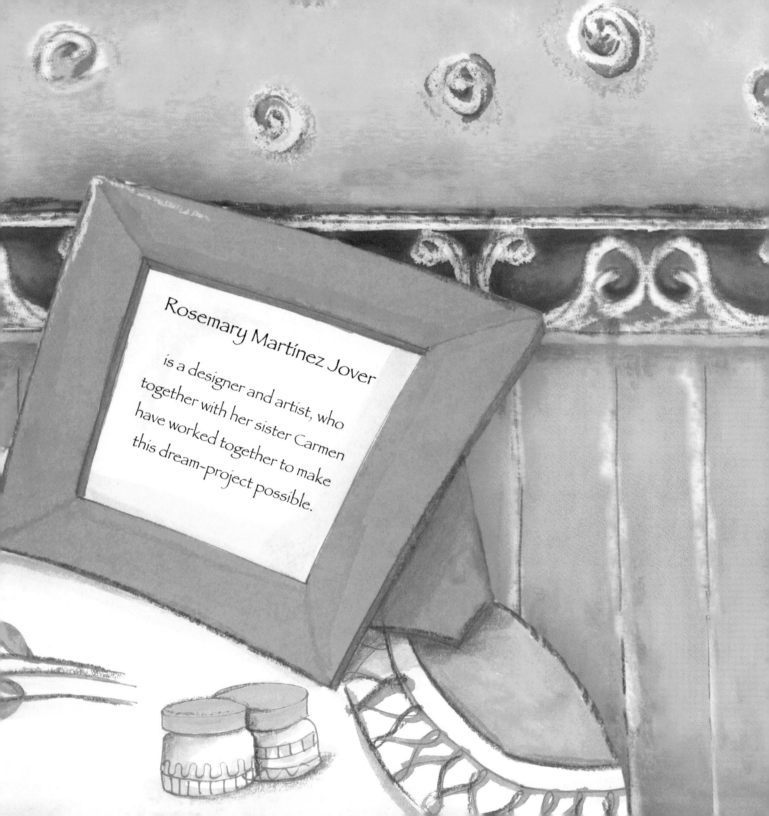

Rosemary Martínez Jover

is a designer and artist, who together with her sister Carmen have worked together to make this dream-project possible.

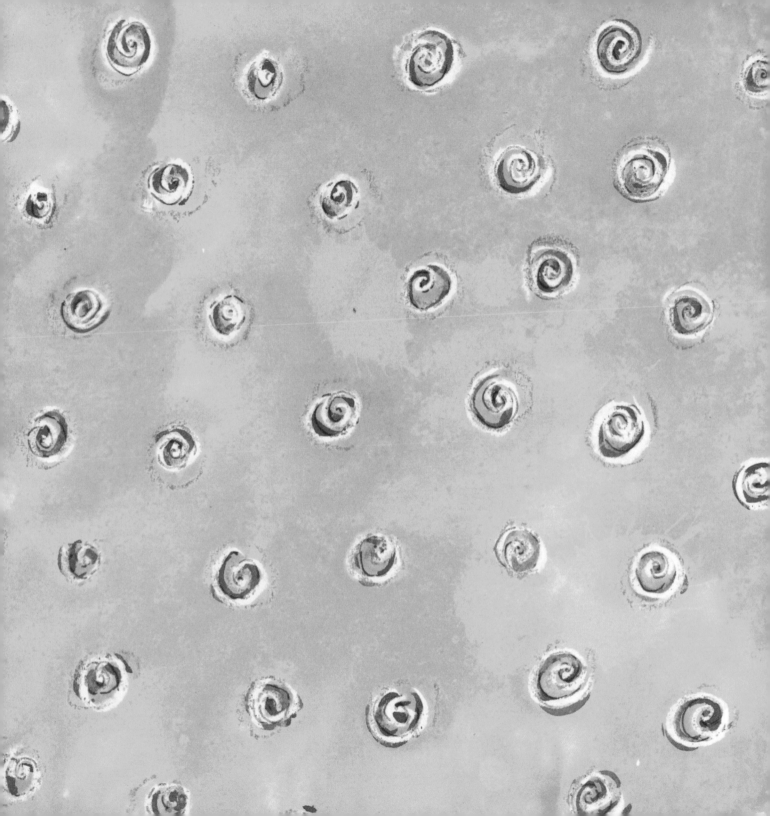

Other Books by
Carmen & Rosemary Martínez Jover

www.carmenmartinezjover.com

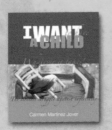

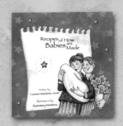

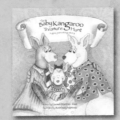

I want to have a child,
Whatever it takes!

Recipes of how babies
are made*

The baby kangaroo
treasure hunt*

* Available in:
English, Español, Français, Italiano,
Português, Svenska, Türkiye, Česky, Русский & עברית

CPSIA information can be obtained
at www.ICGtesting.com
Printed in the USA
LVIC032026310512

283966LV00004BB